Make Your Own Herbal Tinctures

Simple Methods
For Making Your Own Herbal Extracts At Home

By Gabrielle Lilly; MA

Make Your Own Herbal Tinctures
Simple Methods For Making Your Own Herbal Extracts At Home

By Gabrielle Lilly, MA
Practical Healing At Home Series, Book 3

ISBN-13:
978-1976552236

ISBN-10:
1976552230

This book DOES NOT CONTAIN ANY MEDICAL ADVICE, and is not meant to replace necessary medical treatments of any kind.

Making your own herbal extracts is easy to do at home. This is a broad overview of tincture making, and a basic introduction to some commonly used herbs. This book is a good starting point to learn more about using herbs at home. It is my hope that you will take this information as a bridge or leaping point and be inspired to learn more about the art and science of using herbs for healing, cooking, and cosmetics.

There are several ways to make tinctures, and many potential ingredients that can be used. This short book is only introduction to the basic, "simpler's" method, and a short list of some commonly used herbs. I have included a few recipes and ideas for herbal tinctures you can make for yourself and for your family that may help many common ailments. I encourage you to find out more if you are interested in using herbs for healing, cooking, or cosmetics.

I feel inclined to repeat, this information is not meant to take the place of proper medical treatment. None of this is medical advice! Please seek proper medical attention for any serious ailment or disease. Also, these are only a brief introduction, and you are encouraged to experiment and expand on this knowledge to get the best benefits from it for yourself and your loved ones.

Remember, we all are in this together...so be excellent!

About the Author:

Gabrielle Lilly has been practicing the Art and Science of Herbology among family and friends for more than 25 years. She was a NM State Licensed Massage Therapist and Nationally Certified Bodyworker for 10 years and considers herself a novice Certified Herbalist and Aromatherapist.

At the time of writing this, there are no national or state recognized licensure programs for herbology. Gabrielle did receive a certificate of completion for an extensive home-study course in the Art and Science of Herbology, which was written by Master Herbalist Rosemary Gladstar, and which Gabrielle completed in the year 2000.

Gabrielle is an artist, author and musician, with a current special focus on unity, positive alignment, and balancing masculine and feminine energy. She runs a thriving eBay store that sells cosmetic & botanical supplies; such as essential oils, bulk herbs, natural clays and salts, and much more.

You can find her store on eBay at http://stores.ebay.com/Sleeping-Dragons-Company, or find her on Facebook as Gabrielle Angel Dee Lilly.

A note from the author:

Learning about herbs and healing in general is a life-long endeavor. I've had an affinity towards plants and gardening since I was a child. I grew up spending lots of time outdoors. I have been practicing plant identification as long as I can remember. Most of my fondest memories are outside, in trees, gardens, and rivers. Learning to recognize wild onions and asparagus, about which plants I could eat, and which ones were good medicine for certain things, helped me feel more connected with nature, and empowered in my surroundings. I continue this practice today; ever learning, ever growing.

I did not start to study specific herbs and herbal healing deliberately until I was in my 20's, and I was in my late 20's when I decided to take a home-study course on the art and science of herbology. I spent almost two years completing a simple course put together by Rosemary Gladstar (The Art and Science of Herbology), which I highly recommend to anyone who is serious about learning more about herbology and who is looking for a structured course with a little bit of feedback that will not 'break the bank'. **I do not offer any of this information as medical advice or as a substitute for proper medical care and professional supervision when addressing health issues.**

While I don't consider myself a professional herbalist, I do use herbs to help treat myself, and my friends and family for most ailments. I also use them daily in cooking and sometimes as supplements (powdered in capsules). I have been making my own herbal tinctures for friends and family since I became a mother in 1995. I dabbled at first with trying to make standardized tinctures, but I quickly found using a more simple technique commonly called "the simpler's method" was more suitable for me.

My hope is that if you do decide to make your own healing tinctures you will use this information as a starting point and an inspiration to learn more about tinctures and herbal healing in general and about specific herbs. I welcome your feedback and I love to hear about my fellow herbal enthusiasts' experiences with herbs, so please do share any stories you are inspired to share!

Introduction:
What is a tincture?

A tincture is basically an extract of the chemical constituents of a plant or plants, usually made with alcohol and water. Tinctures can also be vinegar or vegetable glycerin based, but most often they are alcohol and water based solutions. Tinctures are not essential oils, though some tinctures do contain some of the volatile essential oils, as well as all the other chemical constituents that are extracted.

Making herbal tinctures at home is easy, and it can be a cost effective way to explore herbal healing and learn more about specific herbs, while also helping to keep your family healthy and happy. Tinctures were once more popular in the medical and pharmaceutical industries, but today tinctures are most popular with herbalists and other complementary or "alternative medicine" practitioners. They are still used in the pharmaceutical industries, and in those cases they are made with precise measurements, set ratios, and then processed with a 'drip method'.

A tincture is basically an extract that lasts. Water can extract some of the chemical parts, or constituents, and water based *infusions* (tea) and *decoctions* make excellent remedies for many ailments. However water based extracts do not last more than 2-3 days before they risk bacteria growth, even when refrigerated, and they take 5-25 minutes to make, which makes them less convenient than tinctures or pills for regular use.

A tincture that is at least 40% alcohol (80 proof) will extract most of the chemical constituents from whatever you put in it, and then keep them relatively the same for many months or years, possibly even decades.

Tinctures are also sometimes made with vinegar or vegetable glycerin. Both of these methods will yield a longer lasting extract than a plain water decoction. Vinegar tinctures will change over time, and obviously, they have a strong vinegar flavor. Glycerin is often preferred for its sweet flavor. Glycerin tinctures are popular for use with children.

The Basic Simpler's Method:

The basic idea is to soak some herbs in alcohol and water until the properties of the herbs are extracted into the alcohol (or vinegar, or glycerin), strain the herbs out, then store the extract for use as needed. Tinctures last longer than powdered herbs. They also can be a convenient and sometimes more effective way to get the healing effects of many herbs.

Alcohol extracts the majority of chemical constituents from most plants. Delicate plant parts, such as flowers and leaves, will be fully extracted, and exhausted of healing properties more quickly than tougher plant parts, like roots and bark. You can tell when most of the chemical constituents have been extracted into the alcohol or glycerin because the herbs will look washed out and lifeless. Some or all the color may be gone from the plant material and extracted into the liquid.

Alcohol tinctures have at least a 2 year shelf life in most cases, making them a practical choice for treatment of many common ailments. Some practitioners (mostly from a more Eastern Medicine persuasion than is common here in the West) will keep tinctures for many years, or even decades; adding fresh or freshly dried herbs to the jar and topping with alcohol as needed. This will result in greater variation of strength, but is still an effective method of tincturing.

If alcohol is a concern, the tincture can be added to hot water or tea, and the alcohol will evaporate out, leaving only the healing properties of the herbs. Those wanting to avoid alcohol more strictly will want to make tinctures with vinegar or vegetable glycerin. Vinegar and glycerin will extract many properties of the herbs, though not as thoroughly as alcohol. Vinegar has a strong flavor to contend with. Glycerin tastes sweet, and often preferred for extracts for children. Elderberries and flowers in glycerin make a fine cough syrup.

Vinegar tinctures have a shorter shelf life than alcohol, but still should last several months. Glycerin tinctures have a longer shelf life than vinegar. However glycerin does not extract therapeutic properties of herbs as thoroughly as the other choices, and technically speaking, the end result is more of a syrup or elixir than a tincture.

Despite the variation of strength inherent in most tinctures, one-eighth to one-quarter teaspoon of tincture is generally considered equivalent to about one cup of herbal tea, or one dose. Tinctures can be made with strict attention to the exact quantities of specific chemical constituents.

Pharmaceutical methods involve strict measurements of chemical content first, then usually a drip-through method of extraction. This results in a more precisely measurably dose of the tincture regarding whatever specific chemicals that are being standardized, but it may lose some of the potential synergistic and energetic properties that this more simple and perhaps more organic method captures.

I will address "the simpler's" method here, as that is the only method I am personally familiar with.

1. First, put dry chopped herbs in a glass jar and cover them with 80 proof (of stronger) alcohol. You can use 90% alcohol (Everclear) and then dilute the tincture with some purified water to no less than 40% alcohol if you desire.

2. Soak them for at least a few weeks, or several months. Shake them daily or at least now and then.

3. Strain or press the herbs out, label your tincture with the date and what is in it, and use the tincture as needed.

Making tinctures with "the simpler's" method results in great potential for variation in strength, so I recommend using a more precise method and educate yourself further if you decide to work with very powerful herbs. Most herbs are relatively safe in small doses such as one would get in a tea or single dose of tincture.

Most commercially available tinctures are formulated and marked for a specific strength, which refers to the ratio of herb and alcohol in the tincture. To get the most precise and accurate measurements, commercial grade tinctures often use almost pure alcohol (190 proof Everclear) and then dilute the tincture to 50:50% alcohol: water after the extraction and straining process is complete.

Everclear is less readily available than 80 proof rum, brandy, and vodka, so most home-remedy makers use one or more of these. I like to use vodka as it has the least flavor, but many prefer brandy or rum for the flavor that it adds. Any ingestible quality grain alcohol of at least 40% alcohol (80 proof) is acceptable for "the simpler's" method, although 100 proof (50%) is a little bit better.

Never use isopropyl rubbing alcohol! It is highly toxic if ingested!

Guidelines for Making Herbal Formulas

Herbal healing sometimes uses single herbs, but more often they are combined for a synergistic effect. The art and science of herbal formulation can be a life-long hobby or take years of intensive study to master. I am certainly NOT a master in this area. When I do 'dabble' with formulas, I always try to keep my blends simple. Of course I also use herbs I am familiar with and know to be safe for myself and my loved ones.

As a general rule of thumb, or starting place, I use a three-point formulation process when I am making a custom formula for a specific complaint or problem. I aim for about 60-75% of my formula to address the main complaint or problem, or desired outcome. About 20-30% of the formula will be supporting herbs, or herbs that address possible negative side effects of the other herbs, such as upsetting the stomach or having a very bad taste. 5-15% will be catalyst herbs, such as ginger, cayenne, hyssop, or cinnamon, that will often help make all the other herbs work more effectively or increase the synergistic effect of all the herbs in the formula.

Obviously, there are many, many herbs that will fit into each category, so in order to choose, you must make other considerations. As a minimum, other considerations include the constitution and of the person the formula is for, as well as the availability and cost of the herbs. There are many other considerations, such as other actions, chemical constituents, potential environmental impact of growing or harvesting, energetics of the herbs, and their synergistic effect with each other. These are beyond the scope of this introduction, though certainly worth mentioning and contemplating.

Many of the formulas I use are very general and safe enough for almost anyone with a normal immune system. Now and then however, I make a specific formula for a loved one to address a specific condition. Here is an overview of how I go about making a formula for a specific person, for a specific complaint: (THIS IS NOT MEDICAL ADVICE, SO PLEASE SEEK PROPER MEDICAL ATTENTION IF YOU HAVE ANY SERIOUS MEDICAL ISSUE!)

- First, I determine the main action I want to make a formula for. For example, I may want something for relaxation, or pain relief, or help slaying asleep, or reducing anxiety, or easing cold symptoms, soothing stomach aches, etc. Whatever the main complaint is will determine the main action I want. If I am treating indigestion, then the main action I want is a carminative or stomachic, which soothe the stomach and aid digestion. If I am treating stomach cramps, then the main action I want is analgesic or anodyne, which relieve pain, and/or an antispasmodic action to stop or decrease the spasms.
- Next I consider the person's constitution or any important factors I need to consider. I often make general tinctures for common ailments like colds, coughs, and stomach aches, where I do not have a

specific person in mind. Other times I make a formula for a specific condition affecting a specific loved one. In those cases it is especially important to consider the person's constitution, habits, and possible allergies when making a formula.

- Then I consider any side effects or possible undesirable effects of the herbs I think I might use. There is always more than one herb that will act on a condition. Many herbs also act on more than one condition. I try to keep my formulas as simple as possible, often even using single herbs instead of formulas.

As a place to start, I try to make my formula so that about 60-75% of the herbal content addresses the main complaint, or issue I am addressing; about 20-30% of the formula will address any related secondary issues or possible side effects; and about 5-15% of the formula is reserved to add a catalyst such as ginger or cayenne. In practice, I also take into account flavor and availability of quality herbs, so the percentages in the formulas I make tend to fluctuate.

I make tinctures with single herbs more often than I make formulas. That way I can combine them as I need or want to. For example, I always keep Elderberry tincture on hand to help combat any cold or flu, and I also try to keep wild cherry bark tincture around for coughs and colds. A good tummy soothing blend is also a necessity in my household. I usually like to keep it simple with Chamomile, Peppermint, Catnip, and Ginger.

Some very simple sample recipes or formulas:

The following outlines are a handful of simple formulas that you can try. As you gain more knowledge about herbs you will see it is easy to make substitutions or variations in these and most other formulas. After you measure your herbs into a glass jar, simply cover them with alcohol, close tightly, shake well, and let time work its magic!

Tummy Soothing Blend:
35% Chamomile
35% Peppermint
15% Yarrow
15% Ginger

Calming Blend
35% Catnip
35% Chamomile
10% Skullcap (optional)
10% Peppermint
10% Cinnamon and/or Ginger

Decongestion Blend
40% Wild Cherry Bark
30% Peppermint
20% Licorice Root
5% Cayenne
5% Ginger

Immunity Booster Blend
25% Elderberry
25% Echinacea Purpurea
20% Elethero (aka "Siberian Ginseng")
20% Yarrow flowers
10% Ginger

Tips, Cautions, and Encouragement

Make sure your herbs are completely covered with alcohol while they soak in the jar. Keep in mind that some herbs may expand considerably while they soak, so add a little more than it takes to cover them initially.

Comfrey root and other herbs that have high mucilage content will need extra room to expand. They may also be harder to strain or press the finished tincture back out of.

The first time I made a single comfrey root tincture, I filled a quart jar about three quarter full with cut comfrey root, filled the jar all the way up with rum, covered it and shook it well. By the next day it had expanded so that I could not shake it very well, so I tried to remove some of it, thinking I would start a second jar and add more alcohol to both jars (which I eventually did succeed in doing). The comfrey root packed itself so tightly that it was surprisingly difficult to get the mixture back out of the jar. I had to use a spoon and a good deal of muscle power, as it had packed itself into a tight, gluey mess! As a result I probably err on the side of caution and may make my tinctures a bit weak sometimes.

I encourage you to experiment and find what herbs and methods work best for you. The art and science of herbology is, as I mentioned, a life-long endeavor. As you begin to use herbs more deliberately in your life; taste them, smell them, touch them, recognize them, you will find they have much to offer. Understanding and using herbs can be a great enhancement to your health on many levels.

Don't be afraid to experiment! Educate yourself about any herb you are going to use, and then try it out. See how it suits you. A great tool for developing a deeper understanding of herbs and your relationship to them is to keep an herb journal. You can write about your experiences with individual herbs as you try them, and if possible, find a picture, or better yet, find some growing outside, and take some notes on what you notice. You will start to notice that plants give us clues about their chemical constituents in their colors, fragrances, shapes, and tastes.

Some Common Herbs You Might Use To Make Tinctures:

The following information is for educational purposes only and is NOT INTENDED AS MEDICAL ADVICE FOR ANY DISEASE!
Please use common sense and seek appropriate medical attention for any medical condition.

Astragalus is a traditional Chinese herb that's used to treat many problems in the body. But it's especially known for helping to boost the body's immunity and to fight viruses – some of the toughest germs around. For a helpful overall boost, astragalus can be combined with ginseng. The two work together to help with problems such as fatigue, lack of appetite, and problems with excessive perspiration. Even used alone, astragalus can be very helpful for improving the body's immunity.

Astralagus is also able to help boost the production of white blood cells in the body. These are the cells that are most responsible for fighting infection. So if you can actually boost the amount of white blood cells in the body, it will be easier for your body to prevent and fight disease. Astralagus may be a very good herb for helping people with immune suppression to help improve immunity. It can help boost white blood cells that are dwindling because of other illnesses or congenital conditions.

Burdock actually has three major benefits: it's an antibacterial agent, an antifungal agent, and it works as a diuretic. As an antibacterial agent, burdock can do many things. First, you can use it topically to treat minor skin problems such as bruises and scrapes. It can also help to speed the healing of burns and protect you from infection.

Burdock can also be used topically on the skin to help treat acne. Acne is actually a tiny bacterial infection under the skin. When you use burdock, you help to kill off the bacteria and give your skin a chance to heal. As an antifungal, burdock is helpful in relieving conditions such as athlete's foot. It can also treat skin irritations like eczema and psoriasis. Some people even use burdock to treat tumors on the skin. It does seem to help treat those tumors and give you long term relief.

Finally, the diuretic action of burdock leaf is also valuable. It can help to relieve pain from rheumatism and arthritis. It can also help to support a healthy kidney function. If you're suffering from bloating and water weight gain, burdock leaf can also help you to get some relief from swelling. Burdock is thought to even help treat diabetes. It supports normal blood function and can help to control your blood sugar.

If you have problems with diarrhea, you'll want to avoid burdock until everything returns to normal. That's because it works as a diuretic and combined with diarrhea could cause you to become dehydrated.

Cascara Sagrada is an herb that's native to the North American continent. Traditionally, it's been used to treat problems with constipation – and that's still its major use. Many Native American tribes used cascara as a laxative in various ways.

Cascara sagrada works as a laxative and is a little bit of a stimulant for the intestines. It's still used today to help treat constipation. If you suffer from chronic constipation, you'll find cascara sagrada particularly helpful. In today's modern diet, many people don't get enough fiber in their diet. Couple that with large amounts of stress, less physical activity, and poor sleeping habits and you often find people who have problems with constipation.

Most people take cascara sagrada bark in fluid extracts or tinctures that are flavored or in the form of pills and powders. Cascara sagrada tea has lost favor because of its bitter flavor.

If you have chronic constipation, you may want to take cascara sagrada daily to help keep your intestines moving. This should also be coupled, of course, with improvements in your diet and moderate exercise. For occasional problems with constipation, you can take cascara sagrada during the duration of the episode. It's a natural way to relieve constipation that won't cause you to have many cramps and doesn't lead to issues with diarrhea as some medicinal laxatives can. It takes about 6-12 hours for cascara sagrada to take effect after the first dose. So be patient once you've begun to use the treatment. Not only does cascara sagrada help to keep your intestines moving, it also helps to tone up the muscles of the large intestine. That means you'll be more likely to have good colon health and tone.

Catnip received it name, because cats like to nip at the plant. It seems to affect them as an aphrodisiac and a euphoric. Catnip doesn't cause any such behavior in humans, but it is particularly beneficial because of its excellent sedative, digestive and nutritional properties.

Like so many other popular botanicals, Catnip also has many excellent nutritional properties, and the leaf of Catnip is highly valued in herbal medicine. The primary chemical constituents of Catnip include essential oils (carvacrol, citronellal, geraniol, nepetol, nepetelactone, pulegone, thymol), iridoids and tannins. It also contains iron, selenium, potassium, manganese, chromium and other nutrients.

Catnip has soothing and relaxing effects on the digestive system, relieving diarrhea, flatulence, indigestion and upset stomach. Catnip contains antispasmodic properties that are said to be useful for treating abdominal and menstrual cramping, as well as chronic coughing. Thought to be excellent for reducing fevers, Catnip's antibiotic and astringent properties are also considered beneficial for treating colds and bronchial infections. Catnip's sedative qualities have also been used to alleviate sleeplessness, insomnia and headaches.

Chamomile is a gentle and highly effective herb known throughout most of the world, and used continually for many centuries. It is a potent yet safe nervine. It is often ingested as a tea or tincture to calm the nervous system and the digestive tract, and is mild enough to be administered to babies with colic.

Chamomile is soothing to irritated skin and membranes, and so is often found in lotions and hair products. Other studies illuminate this plant's potential to assist in healing wounds and soothing gastrointestinal conditions.

Chamomile is slightly bitter, sweet, and generally considered pleasant tasting. It is a tonic, adodyne, carminative, sedative, stomachic, laxative, diaphoretic, emmenagogic, and anxiolytic. It has been shown in scientific studies to promote wound healing when applied topically. Chamomile has a reputation of being the rare combination of both a bitter digestive tonic and a relaxant, or sedative, meaning that it has both the ability to tone the digestive organs and at the same time relax the nervous system.

Elderberries and Elder Flowers have been used for thousands of years to treat problems that arise from inflammation. These are flowers and berries from the elder tree. The tree has an interesting history. It was once believed that Elder Mother lived inside the tree. No one would cut down the tree because they were afraid to make her angry.

Elder flowers and berries can also help keep your digestive system regular. Elder may help with any intestinal problem you have. Whether it's diarrhea or constipation, elderflower is the right treatment. Strangely it can work for both conditions.

If you're suffering from fever, elderflower can help you to get relief. It causes you to sweat profusely and that allows the heat to be reduced. Its ability to make you sweat can also help you to have fewer problems with toxins in the blood. Elderflower encourages the removal of toxins from the blood and leaves you with fewer problems such as arthritis.

If you're suffering from problems with your respiratory system, you'll find that elderflower and elderberries can bring relief. You'll benefit from this plant's ability to work as an expectorant. That means it can thin the mucous that's causing your problem and allow your coughs to be more productive. While you may cough more at first, your coughs will be more productive. That means that you'll actually be clearing out your lungs.

Elderflowers and berries can reduce your problems with mucous from upper respiratory infections, and also help you with the mucous that comes from seasonal allergies and hay fever. It can boost your immune system so you'll have fewer problems with colds and other illnesses that get passed around.

If you have dry skin, elderflower can also soothe it and bring relief. You'll have more moisture and less irritation when you apply a cream containing the herb directly to your skin. Elder flower is a good all around herb that helps to keep you healthy and strong and can still be used to treat specific conditions. It's also a typically safe herb to use. Elderberry tincture is one of my favorites to keep in the kitchen and add an extra boost to nearly any hot tea, especially during cold and flu season.

Fennel may be something you've used for cooking. It provides a flavorful addition to salads and to many different recipes. Fennel is more than just a tasty treat. As with many popular cooking herbs, it has soothing carminative properties, and can help aid digestion.

Fennel is helpful for menstrual and digestive disorders. If you're feeling bloated, gassy, or have an upset stomach, fennel can help bring you some relief.

It can also be used as a companion to laxatives. While some laxatives can cause uncomfortable intestinal cramping, fennel actually can relieve cramps and allow you to feel comfortable.

When you have problems with your skin, such as minor irritations and burns, a fennel solution can bring soothing relief. Fennel can even be used in an infusion to treat problems like conjunctivitis, an inflammation of the lining of the eye.

For women who are breastfeeding, fennel can be used to prevent mastitis. It actually helps to release breast milk and allow you to nurse your baby productively and with more comfort. Chewing on a piece of fennel can also help to improve your breath and settle your stomach after a heavy meal.

Science has shown that fennel works as an anti-inflammatory and an anti-spasmodic. It relieves muscle tension and cramping and soothes inflammatory problems in the body. It also contains stimulants that help to break up mucous in the respiratory tract and relieve congestion.

Keeping fennel in your cabinet will help you to be prepared for problems with menstrual or intestinal cramping. If you're a nursing mother, you can also benefit from the effects it will have on your breast milk. It's a great way to prevent the painful infection of mastitis.

Fennel seed tincture is a good main staple for the medicine or kitchen cabinet, as it can be used alone or in a formula to help soothe the action of other herbs. Fennel is generally considered safe to use with children and elderly people.

Gentian is native to Europe and Asia, but can be purchased anywhere in the world today. When it comes to stomach upset, most people reach for a bottle of pink liquid to relieve their symptoms. But there's another way you can actually treat your upset stomach naturally.

Gentian is thought to work so well because it is a bitter herb that stimulates the nervous system to produce saliva and gastric juices. This in turn actually helps to stimulate the appetite. It also promotes the normal function of the digestive system. When everything is moving properly, you'll have fewer complaints.

If you're suffering from loss of appetite due to an illness, gentian may be exactly what you need to keep your appetite stimulated. You may also find that it can be useful if you have an upset stomach or even intestinal illness such as diarrhea and cramping. When your liver isn't functioning at full par, you can also count on gentian to help detoxify the body and stimulate the liver.

If you have a fever, gentian can help to lower it and give you relief and comfort. In addition, gentian can also be used to treat anemia by stimulating red blood cell production. This is particularly good for someone suffering from a low red blood cell count. Gentian can help restore energy and vitality. You can take gentian several ways. It can be used as an infusion or a tincture, depending on what you need it to do. When taking gentian, follow the manufacturer's instructions so that you don't take too much or too little.

Gentian is like having a broad spectrum of stomach medicines in your cabinet. Make sure to keep a supply of it in your medicine cabinet for those times when your stomach doesn't agree with what you've eaten or your appetite is diminished. And if you tend to have anemic blood, taking gentian regularly can prevent you from having fatigue.

Ginger Root is most commonly known for its effectiveness as a digestive aid. Chinese ships carried pots of Ginger aboard when on long sea voyages to prevent scurvy and sea sickness, and a Chinese folk remedy recommends rubbing the cut root of the plant on the scalp to stop hair loss. Ginger Root has also been used for centuries in Chinese herbal medicine for the positive effects it has on the body. Ginger's sweet taste has made it a popular herb, and it is found today in ginger ale, breads, candies and tonics.   By increasing the production of digestive fluids Ginger can enhance the effectiveness of herbal combinations.

Ginger may help to relieve indigestion, gas pains, diarrhea and stomach cramping. The primary known constituents of Ginger Root include gingerols, zingibain, bisabolenel, oleoresins, starch, essential oil (zingiberene, zingiberole, camphene, cineol, borneol), mucilage and protein. Ginger Root is also used to treat nausea related to both motion sickness and morning sickness and is said to be even more effective than Dramamine® in curbing motion sickness, without causing drowsiness.

Ginger's anti-inflammatory properties are thought to help relieve pain and reduce inflammation associated with arthritis, rheumatism and muscle spasms. Ginger's therapeutic properties are believed to effectively stimulate circulation of the blood, removing toxins from the body, cleansing the bowels and kidneys, and nourishing the skin.

Other uses for Ginger Root include the treatment of asthma, bronchitis and other respiratory problems by loosening and expelling phlegm from the lungs. Ginger Root may also be used to help break fevers by warming the body and increasing perspiration.

Contraindications:

People taking blood thinners (Coumadin, aspirin, etc.) should avoid Ginger, and the herb should be avoided for two weeks prior to elective surgery. Pregnant women who use Ginger for morning sickness should not take large amounts (many times the recommended dose) nor use it for prolonged periods without consulting a physician. Ginger increases bile production and should not be used by people with gallstones or gallbladder disease unless supervised by a doctor.

Guarana is a vine that grows in the Brazilian rain forest. Tribes all along the Amazon have used it for thousands of years to improve the health of their people. Guarana was a staple of the Brazilian diet and could be found in soda, syrups, candies, and other products since the early 1900s. Today, millions of people in Brazil still use guarana as a tonic herb that improves their vitality and gives them energy.

Guarana is known for its ability to purify the blood and to help reduce fatigue. It also has antioxidant properties that help it to fight the aging process. It has even been suggested that guarana is a reason that Brazilians are so beautiful.

If you're interested in using guarana, you'll be thrilled to know that it can also be used to treat digestive system issues such as diarrhea, gas, and stomach upset. In addition, it can be used to help suppress the appetite and aid in weight loss.

If you're suffering from fatigue and general low energy, taking guarana can help to put some pep in your step. It's also known to help make the heart stronger and to increase sexual performance. Guarana does contain a great deal of caffeine and tannins. This is probably the reason it works to stimulate the brain and the rest of the nervous system. It also works to thin the blood and provide energy that way.

It's also important to make sure that you don't combine guarana with certain drugs such as MAO inhibitors that work to thin the blood. Guarana can interact with some medications and should not be combined with them. Talk to your healthcare provider to find out if guarana is safe for you. Guarana should also not be taken with appetite suppressants or supplements containing ephedra. Together it will act to speed the heart up too much. Make sure to read labels before taking guarana.

If you're looking for an overall supplement that can

help to increase your energy and decrease your appetite, guarana may be the right choice for you. You can stock up on powdered or tinctured guarana to keep in your cupboard. Taking it as part of your daily routine can help to keep you looking and feeling young.

Hops: You probably know that hops are one of the major ingredients in the popular beverage beer. It's a plant that's been used to brew the beverage for centuries. However, hops can be used for much more than making an alcoholic liquid. In fact, you'll wonder why you didn't know more about hops before.

Dried hops can be used for a variety of things. For example, if you're having problems with inflammation of a joint or other area of the body, you can create a poultice of dried hops. When you apply it directly to the affected area, you'll enjoy soothing relief. In addition, hops can be put in a sachet made of cheesecloth or old nylons and placed under your pillow. This will help you to fall asleep and have sweet dreams if you're suffering from insomnia.

If you suffer from menstrual cramps that sometimes seem unbearable, hops can also help you to find relief. The plant works to fight muscle spasms that cause the painful cramps. In addition, it can fight spasms in the respiratory system that cause asthma.

This work with muscle spasms extends to the digestive system as well. If you suffer from indigestion or irritable bowel syndrome, hops can bring relief by relaxing the muscles of the digestive system. In addition, hops can be a good treatment for increasing your appetite if you've lost it due to illness.

Hops can be used in many forms such as infusions, liquid extracts, tinctures, oils, and tablets. You'll need to follow the manufacturer's instructions before taking it to make sure you get the dosage correct. You may also find that hops are an ingredient in teas that are designed to help you sleep at night.

One word to the wise, hops can actually cause some skin irritation if you handle the plant directly. It can cause dermatitis and eye irritation if you get it in your eyes. In addition, some people have an allergy to hops. Make sure to handle hops with care so you can avoid these irritations and complications. Used correctly, hops can be a great addition to your herbal regimen. You may wonder how you ever lived without it.

Licorice Root not only tastes great, but it's a beneficial herb as well! Licorice helps cleanse the colon, supports lung health and promotes adrenal gland function. Licorice is a common ingredient in throat-soothing herbal supplements, and its natural sweetness makes it a favorite flavor in herbal teas and many food products.

Ancient cultures on every continent have used Licorice Root, included recorded use by the Egyptians in the third century B. C. The Egyptians and the Greeks also recognized the herb's benefits in treating coughs and lung disease, and it was so highly valued in ancient Egypt that even King Tutankhamen was buried with a supply.

The most common medical use for Licorice Root is for treating upper respiratory ailments including coughs, hoarseness, sore throat and bronchitis. This herb is thought to be as effective as codeine, and possibly safer, when used as a cough suppressant. Rhizomes in Licorice have a high mucilage content which, when mixed with water or used in cough drops, sooths irritated mucous membranes. The use of Licorice also has an expectorant effect which increases the secretion of the bronchial glands.

Today, herbal preparations containing Licorice Root are used to treat stomach and intestinal ulcers, lower acid levels and coat the stomach wall with a protective gel. Rarely used alone, Licorice is a common component of many herbal teas as a mild laxative, a diuretic and a carminitive for flatulence.

It has also been thought to relieve rheumatism and arthritis, regulate low blood sugar, and may be effective for Addison's disease (under the doctor's care). The Root extract produces mild estrogenic effects and it has proven useful in treating symptoms of menopause, regulating menstruation and relieving menstrual cramps.

The constituent, glycyrrhizin, is fifty times sweeter than sugar, making Licorice a widely used ingredient in the food industry. The distinctive flavor of Licorice Root makes it a popular additive to baked confections, liqueurs, ice cream and candies. It is also widely used in other medicines to mask bitter tastes and also to prevent pills from sticking together.

Licorice has also been used in poultices for treatment of dermatitis and skin infections. It helps to open the pores and is used in combination with other cleansing and healing herbs as an emollient. Ninety percent of the Licorice imported into America is used to flavor tobacco, and other uses of Licorice include cattle and horse feed.

Contraindications:

Pregnant women, diabetics and those with high blood pressure should avoid this herb. People suffering from heart disease should not use Licorice unless under a physician's care. According to the German Commission E monograph, Licorice supplements are contraindicated in people with liver and kidney disorders, and thus, people with kidney disease, gallbladder disease and cirrhosis should avoid this herb. Large doses of Licorice may induce sodium retention and potassium depletion and can lead to hypertension and edema. Use of Licorice should be done under the supervision of a health care provider or qualified practitioner.

The herb is not meant for long term use and should not be taken for more than seven days in a row. Long-term intake of products containing more than one gram of glycyrrhizin (the amount in approximately ten grams of root, which is far in excess of the daily dosage recommended by this product) is the usual amount required to cause these types of effects. Do not take Licorice without speaking with your physician if you take the heart medication, Digoxin (Lanoxicaps®, Lanoxin®, Lanoxin Pediatric®) or prescription diuretics (which may lead to loss of potassium, which may cause fatigue, muscle cramps, headaches, swelling, increase urination, breathlessness or high blood pressure). Other possible drug interactions with any Licorice product include potentiation of anticoagulants and possible interference with hormonal therapy due to estrogenic activity of

Licorice (including decreased testosterone and birth control pills).

Prickly Ash Bark: Long before European settlers came to the United States, prickly ash bark was used to treat a wide variety of problems. However, its most common use was that of toothache relief. In fact, the prickly ash tree is often called the "toothache tree" because the bark works so well at improving the condition.

It works so well at helping toothache pain go away because it stimulates the circulation. When an area of the body has improved circulation, it actually helps healing to occur more quickly. That's because having more blood moving through the area allows the blood to deliver more healing nutrients and it allows the blood to take the toxins away. Prickly ash bark works very well at improving circulation in a specific, targeted area.

While it was once used primarily for toothaches – and still works quite well – it's now used mainly to treat rheumatism or arthritis. It provides relief because it stimulates circulation in those areas and helps to soothe inflammation. It can also be used directly on the skin to treat open sores.

If you suffer from conditions that arise from poor circulation, prickly ash can help you to get relief. Taken internally, prickly ash bark can actually help your circulation to improve in all of the limbs. If you're tired of having limbs that fall asleep and having difficulty with healing in those areas, you'll appreciate the benefits of prickly ash bark.

Finally, if you have problems with your digestive

system, prickly ash bark may be the perfect solution. It will work to treat diarrhea and can help to relieve gas. If you have a problem with irritable bowel syndrome, or even just indigestion, this may be a good remedy for you.

Prickly Ash Bark can be taken as a tincture or decoction. It can also be purchased in commercially produced tablets. Finally, you can use it in the form of a lotion to help relieve skin irritations or to improve circulation. It will be absorbed through the skin in this form.

Prickly ash bark shouldn't be used if you're pregnant, nor should it be used if you have a sensitive stomach. Like many herbs that affect circulation, it can cause some stomach upset. However, most people are able to tolerate prickly ash bark well and find that it helps them with their condition. There's no need to suffer with poor circulation or arthritis when there's a simple solution to keep you healthy and strong.

Peppermint is more than just a candy flavor. This herb promotes healthy digestion by soothing and comforting the stomach. Peppermint is frequently used in herbal teas and Capsules. The essential oil of this plant contains menthol, which also displays healthful powers, and is often found in throat-soothers and topical vapor rubs.

Mint is one of the most ancient of all medicinal herbs. Ancient Athenians would rub the leaves of mint on their arms to improve their endurance, and both Greeks and Romans crowned themselves with Peppermint at their feasts and adorned their tables with its sprays. They also flavored their sauces and their wines with its essence.

Peppermint is an excellent carminative, having a relaxing effect on the muscles of the digestive system, combating flatulence and stimulating bile and digestive juice flow. It is used to relieve intestinal colic, flatulent dyspepsia and associated conditions. The volatile oil in Peppermint acts as a mild anesthetic to the stomach wall, which allays feelings of nausea and the desire to vomit. This herb has long been known to relieve nausea and vomiting associated with pregnancy, as well as travel sickness.

Peppermint is also used in the treatment of ulcerative conditions of the bowel. It is a traditional treatment for fevers, colds and influenza. Where headaches are associated with indigestion, Peppermint may help. As a nervine, it eases anxiety and tension. In cases of painful menstrual periods, the herb relieves the pain and eases associated tension. Externally, it is used to relieve itching, inflammation and a variety of respiratory conditions. Peppermint oil is also a great expectorant.

Contraindications:

Pregnant and nursing women should not take Peppermint without consulting a physician. Peppermint may aggravate hiatal hernia. Those who suffer from gallbladder disorders, gallstones or blockage of the bile duct, or those who take heartburn medication (cisapride, etc.) should not take Peppermint without consulting a physician. Do not exceed dosage (many time the recommended amount), and it is also recommended to take a few days' break after two weeks' continual use. Peppermint may interfere with absorption of iron.

Red Clover has been used for centuries as a fine expectorant and an analgesic and is also a wonderful blood purifier and cleanser. This is another herb I like to keep a neat tincture of for frequent use by itself or in nearly any hot tea.Red Clover is a vitally nutritional, mineral-rich herb that is used as a great tonic for overall good health. Herbalists have long prized this herb for its traditional use as a blood purifier, expelling toxins from the bloodstream. Primary chemical constituents of Red Clover include phenolic glycosides (salicylic acid), essential oil (methyl salicylate), sitosterol, genistein, flavonoids, coumarins, cyanogenic glycosides, silica, choline and lecithin. Red Clover also contains vitamin A, C, B-complex, calcium, chromium, iron and magnesium.

Red Clover is one of the most useful remedies for children with skin problems, and because it is mild, it makes an excellent nutritional supplement for children. The expectorant and antispasmodic action give this remedy a role in the treatment of coughs and bronchitis, but especially in whooping cough, dry cough and colds.

Red Clover also increases the production of mucus and urine flow, helping relieve irritation and inflammation of the urinary tract. As a digestive aid, Red Clover stimulates the production of digestive fluids and bile. It is also said to relieve constipation and help soothe inflammation of the bowel, stomach and intestines. Red Clover contains easily-absorbed calcium and magnesium that are thought to tone and relaxe the nervous system, relieving tension due to stress and the associated headaches, which are further relieved by the silicic acid content. Clinical evidence shows that there is a basis for its long-standing tradition in treating malignant disease, and its antimicrobial properties are said to be effective against tuberculosis.

For women, Red Clover is quite special. It contains stilbene, which is believed to stimulate eostrogenic activity, thus possibly increasing fertility and reducing "hot flashes" experienced by women during menopause. It also supports the uterus with its vitamin content, and the high protein content nourishes the whole body. There is also an alkalizing effect, which is believed to improve vaginal and uterine acid/alkaline balance.

Rehmannia root is an herb you may not have used before, but it has many uses for the body that can help you to feel healthier, happier, and revitalized. It has positive effects on the blood, liver, and women's health. It's one herb may want to have at the ready in your supply.

Rehmannia root is used extensively in Chinese Medicine as a tonic, and to help strengthen the liver. It can actually be used as a companion to licorice root to treat hepatitis – a viral disease that doesn't have many treatment options in Western medicine. But even if you don't suffer from hepatitis, this herb could help you to have better liver function. It will help to remove toxins from the liver, which can assist you in a variety of ways.

In addition to lowering your blood pressure and cholesterol, there's some scientific evidence that rehmannia root can help you to control blood sugar. This can help to prevent the onset of type II diabetes and can even help to control it once you've been diagnosed.

Some new research also shows that rehmannia root can help to support you throughout the process of menopause. It can help to stimulate hormones in the body and prevent problems such as hot flashes and bone loss. This is a great supplement for someone who wants to avoid the dangers of hormone replacement therapy, but doesn't want to fight the symptoms of menopause.

If you have a fever, rehmannia root can also help you to get your body temperature back to normal. It actually helps to cool the body and allow you to get back to normal quickly. It works so well with this because it works as a diuretic. Rehmannia has long been used as a tonic that helps strengthen the body and provide overall health and wellness.

Schizandra is an herb that is particularly helpful for someone who's recovering from a serious illness. It can help to restore your normal health and vitality and give you what you need to improve your energy levels. Many people know the fatigue that can occur when you've been sick for several days and even weeks or months. In order to get you back on your feet faster, you may want to try schizandra.

When it comes to the liver, using schizandra can help the liver to work properly. It helps to remove toxins from the body and can even be a help for people who suffer from hepatitis. When your liver is functioning properly, you'll immediately find that you have more energy and even your eyes will look brighter.

If you're suffering from a cold or other type of respiratory infection, schizandra can help to loosen the tightness in your chest. It will actually thin the mucus so that you can have more productive coughs and get the thick secretions out of your body. People who suffer from chronic skin conditions will find that schizandra provides relief. It can help to soothe the inflammation and irritation that comes from psoriasis or eczema. It can also relieve pain.

If you're having problems with sex drive or sexual function, you may find that schizandra is the perfect solution. It helps the sexual organs to function properly so that you have the drive and stamina you desire. If you find yourself having difficulty with stress, concentration, or anxiety, schizandra can help you to focus better, and ease your anxiety and stress. It is also said to help improve memory.

To use schizandra, you'll want to take a decoction or tincture of it 3 times a day. This will provide you with all the herb you need to experience improved health. If you've recently suffered from an illness, this is one of the fastest ways to get back on your feet.

Stevia Leaf has been used for centuries as a natural, sugar-free sweetener. Stevia Leaf has also been employed for its antibacterial properties, and is believed by some to be of help in preventing diabetes. Stevia is a safe, all-natural alternative to artificial sweeteners and refined sugar in the diet. It has been used for centuries by native Indians in Paraguay, and consumed safely in massive quantities for the past twenty years. Stevia has also been used for alleviating bleeding gums, sore throats and cold sores due to its mild antibacterial functions. It has also been shown to inhibit the development of plaque and aid in the prevention of cavities.

There have also been some claims that Stevia functions as an antidiabetic agent. Since Stevia does not break down when it is heated, it can be used in foods that are baked or cooked; however, because it does not caramelize, brown or crystallize like sugar does, meringues and caramel may be difficult to make. The refined Stevia extracts are considered to be calorie-free and do not raise blood sugar levels. Whereas the raw herbal form of Stevia contains nearly one hundred identified phytonutrients and volatile oils, Stevia extracts contain negligible nutritive benefits.

Uva ursi has been used as a diuretic and urinary antiseptic for more than 1,000 years by cultures as widely separated as the Chinese and American Indians. Today it is an ingredient in most herbal diuretics and urinary remedies and many weight-loss formulas. Even herbal conservative Varro Tyler, Ph.D., calls it "a modestly effective urinary antiseptic and diuretic."

The Roman physician Galen used uva ursi's astringent leaves to treat wounds and stop bleeding. Still, this herb was largely ignored by Western Herbalists until the 13th century, when Marco Polo reported Chinese physicians using it as a diuretic to treat kidney and urinary problems. Polo's famous travelogue repopularized uva ursi in Europe as a urinary and kidney remedy.

Uva ursi's association with the kidney was

strengthened by the medieval Doctrine of Signatures - the idea that a plant's physical appearance revealed its healing virtues. The herb grew in rocky, gravelly places, and at the time kidney stones were called gravel. In the urinary tract, the arbutin in uva ursi is chemically transformed into an antiseptic chemical, hydroquinone, according to several studies. In addition, the herb contains diuretic chemicals, including ursolic acid, powerful astringents (tannins), and a chemical that helps promote the growth of healthy new cells, allantoin.

Herbal weight loss formulas typically contain diuretics. Uva ursi is the diuretic most often used. Because they boost urine production, diuretics temporarily eliminate some water weight. Weight loss using diuretics almost always invariably returns. Weight control experts do not recommend diuretics. The key to permanent weight control includes a low-fat, high fiber diet, and regular aerobic exercise.

The Food and Drug Administration lists uva ursi as an herb of "undefined safety." For otherwise healthy nonpregnant, nonnursing adults, uva ursi is considered relatively safe in amounts typically recommended.
Uva usri often turns urine a dark green. Do not become alarmed.
Uva ursi should be used in medicinal amounts only in consultation with your doctor.

Valerian root is well known for its ability to help one go to sleep at night, valerian has been used for thousands of years as a sleep aid. And even though there are many products on the market that improve sleep, none come close to the natural effects of valerian root.

Valerian is a plant that is native to Europe. The root of the plant is used in herbal medicine and must be at least two years old before it's unearthed and used by humans for medicinal purposes. It's used to help slow down the body in many ways and provides relief for several problems. For example, if someone is having problems sleeping at night, valerian root can be prescribed to aid in sleep. It's one of the best treatments you'll find as a sleep aid in modern times.

You can also use valerian root to treat problems with stress and anxiety. While it's best known as a sedative used for sleeping, it can also be mild enough to be used to fight anxiety. When you take the appropriate amount of valerian root, you'll feel stress melt away. Muscle tension that's often caused from stress and overworked muscles can also be combated with valerian. It helps to relax the muscles and relieve the pain and tension that comes from too much stress on the muscles.

If you have high blood pressure, particularly due to anxiety, valerian root can also help to return your blood pressure to normal. It helps to fight the physical effects of anxiety on the body and leaves you with sweet relief. Unlike many prescription tranquilizers and sedatives, valerian root is not addictive. You won't find yourself in the position of relying completely on it to relax and sleep at night. It will simply act as an aid in relaxing the muscles so that you can drift off to a peaceful sleep. Even though it's been around a long time, it's still one of the most effective ways to catch some sleep.

Valerian root can be taken in the form of a tincture

and it can be used in the form of a decoction. You can also find valerian in the form of tablets and capsules. While it doesn't pose a dangerous threat because of addiction, valerian root will make you drowsy. You shouldn't operate a vehicle or heavy machinery while using it and you should never combine it with another sleep aid.

Vitex is a plant that's native to the Mediterranean region of the world. It's been used for thousands of years to have an effect on hormones and has even been called "chaste berry" for its ability to help control sexual feelings. There are many stories of monks using it to fight their natural sex drive. For many years, vitex has been an herb that was used to help people remain chaste. But modern research has shown that it does much more than keep people from acting on sexual urges. In fact, it can actually be a major benefit to your reproductive health. Take a look at what vitex can do for women.

If you suffer from problems such as irritability and depression due to hormonal changes in your menstrual cycle, vitex could be the cure you've been looking for. It actually helps to control the symptoms of PMS and relieves the moodiness as well as the physical bloating and discomfort that go along with the syndrome. And if you're dealing with hormonal imbalances that cause irregular periods and mood swings, you'll find that vitex can help to straighten out the body. It will naturally regulate the hormones so that you don't find your moods riding on a pendulum. You'll also find that your period will become more predictable and regulated. Don't expect vitex to work overnight. Just like many hormonal treatments it takes about 90 days to get the full effect. Don't give up on it after a month or even two. Give it a solid three months to make a difference in your hormonal balance.

You can take vitex as a tincture daily in order to get the best benefit. The recommended dosage is 40 drops a day added to water. When you continue this program for several months, you'll find that gradually your hormones will become regulated. Vitex is a great alternative to taking artificial hormones that can cause more problems than they cure.

Yarrow has been used to stop bleeding both internally and externally for centuries. Yarrow is also thought to alleviate inflammation, reduce fevers, stimulate the appetite and encourage sweating, while expelling toxins from the body. Yarrow's astringent properties are especially helpful in stopping nosebleeds, excessive menstruation and diarrhea. Yarrow's effects are mostly astringent. Yarrow nutritionally supports mucus membranes. It is closely related to chamomile, both botanically and chemically. Yarrow also contains fairly high amounts of selenium, potassium, vitamins A, C, E, F and K.

Having a variety of effects on the body, Yarrow is believed to alleviate inflammation, reduce fevers, stimulate the appetite and encourage sweating, thus expelling toxins from the body. Yarrow's astringent properties are especially helpful in stopping nosebleeds, excessive menstruation and diarrhea. Yarrow is also thought to relieve muscle spasms, arthritis and indigestion. Yarrow helps to relax peripheral blood vessels, thereby helping to improve circulation. The constituents, achilletin and achilleine, are said to aid in blood coagulation. Yarrow contains several anti-inflammatory and pain-relieving constituents, such as azulene and salicylic acid.

Contraindications:

Pregnant or nursing women should not use Yarrow, as it is a uterine stimulant, nor should women with heavy periods or pelvic inflammatory disease. Continued or long-term use of Yarrow may cause skin irritation and/or allergic reactions. If so, discontinue its use. Yarrow may produce photosensitivity. If using Yarrow to treat wounds, be sure to clean the affected area first, as the herb can stop blood flow so quickly that it may seal in dirt or other contaminants. People with gallstones should avoid its use. Yarrow may cause severe allergic skin rashes when applied topically.

Useful definitions & Terminology:
The following is a starter list of brief definitions for common medical terms often used when describing herbs and their healing properties:

Adaptogen: An agent that causes adaptive reactions and increases resistance to stress. Adaptogens enable the body to deal with and recover from stress and disease. They appear to increase SNIR (state of non-specifically increased resistance) in the human body, protecting against diverse stresses. Adaptogens usually help produce suitable adjustments in the body. They tend to normalize body functions. When the job is completed, they are eliminated or incorporated into the body without side effects. Adaptogens generally work by strengthening the immune system, nervous system and/or glandular system.

Alterative: Sometimes called blood cleaners, an alterative helps to gradually and favorably alter the course of an ailment or condition. An alterative helps to alter the process of nutrition and excretion and restore normal bodily function. It also acts to cleanse and stimulate the efficient removal of waste products from the system.

Analgesic: Substance that relieves pain by acting as a nervine, antiseptic, antibiotic, antispasmodic or counter irritant.

Anesthetic (local): An agent that reduces pain in an area by desensitizing the nerves. Deadens sensation.

Anodyne: Pain relieving.

Antioxidant: Compound that prevents destructive, free radical or oxidative damage to tissues or cells.

Antipyretic (also called **Febrifuge** or **Refrigerant**): A substance that reduces fever and cools the body.

Anti-rheumatic: An agent that eases the discomfort of or prevents rheumatism, a condition marked by inflammation and pain in the joints and muscles.

Antiseptic: A substance that destroys bacteria and prevents infections. Also helps to prevent tissue degeneration.

Antispasmodic: A "relaxant" or "nervine" that relieves or prevents involuntary muscle contractions or "spasms," such as those occurring in epilepsy, painful menstruation or intestinal cramping.

Anxiety: A condition marked by apprehension of danger and dread, accompanied by nervous restlessness, tension, increased heart rate and shortness of breath.

Aperient: Mild laxative without purging.

Aperitive: Herbs that stimulate the appetite.

Aphrodisiac: Agent that stimulates sexual desire or potency.

Aromatic: Substance containing volatile, essential oils that aid digestion and relieve gas.

Astringent: A substance that contracts, tightens and binds tissues and diminishes (or arrests) internal and external secretions. Can be used to check bleeding and diarrhea.

Ayurvedic: Traditional (and ancient) system of medicine in India. (literally, "A Science of Life").

Bitter: A plant product (often aromatic) that is used as a tonic and stimulates secretions of the digestive tract and encourages appetite.

Carminative: Agent that relieves intestinal gas pain and distension by expelling gases from the stomach and bowels. Also promotes peristalsis (contraction and relaxing of bowel). Frequently improves digestion.

Cathartic: A laxative. (1) Aperient is a mild laxative that promotes evacuation of the bowels by action on alimentary canal and (2) purgative that causes copious, rapid evacuation of the bowel and generally used to treat stubborn constipation in adults.

Contraindications: Any factor that makes it unwise to pursue a certain line of treatment.

Decoction: A water extract of bark or roots prepared at a low boil for ten to twenty minutes.

Demulcent: Mucilaginous substance that acts to soothe and relieve inflammation. Softens and soothes damaged or inflamed tissues.

Diaphoretic: Substance that produces perspiration and elimination through the skin.

Digestive: Substance that aids digestion, usually by providing enzymes from various sources.

Diuretic: Substance that increases and promotes the secretion and flow of urine.

Emetic: Substance that causes vomiting.

Emmenagogue: Substance that promotes and stimulates menstruation.

Expectorant: A substance that loosens and expels mucous secretions and phlegm from the respiratory systems and air passages. Promotes the thinning and ejection of mucus or exudates from the lungs, bronchi and trachea.

Febrifuge (also called **Antipyretic** and **Refrigerant**): Agent that lessens fever and cools the body.

Infusion: A preparation made by steeping the plant material in hot water for twenty minutes, generally making it stronger than tea.

Nervine: A substance that calms and soothes the nerves and reduces tension and anxiety. A tonic for the nervous system that eases stress, nervous disorders and nourishes the nerves.

Nutritive: Nourishes and builds body tissues.

Purgative: A substance that promotes bowel movement and increased intestinal peristalsis.

Relaxant: A substance that relaxes nerves and muscles and reduces tension, especially muscular tension.

Restorative: Substance that renews health and strength and is effective in the regaining of normal physiological activity.

Rubefacient: Herbs that, when applied to the skin, stimulate circulation in that area of normal physiological activity.

Stimulant: An herb that increases the activity or efficiency of a system or organ - acts more rapidly than a tonic herb.

Stomachic: An agent that relieves gastric disorders. It tones and gives strength to the stomach, helps digestion and improves the appetite.

Tannin: An astringent phenolic plant constituent.

Tonic: A substance that exerts a gentle strengthening effect on the body. Designed to restore enfeebled function and to promote vigor and a sense of well-being. Tonic herbs restore and strengthen individual organs and the entire system.

Uterostimulant: Substance that stimulates the uterus.

Vasoconstrictor: An agent that narrows blood vessel openings, restricting the flow of blood through them.

Vasodilator: An agent that causes relaxation of blood vessels.

Vermicide: A medicine that kills intestinal worms.

Vermifuge (also called **Anthelmintic**): A substance that destroys and expels intestinal worms.

Vulnerary: A substance that arrests bleeding in wounds and prevents tissue degeneration.

References:

- Foster, S. Herbal Renaissance. Utah: Peregine Smith Books; 1984.
- Hartung, T. *Growing 101 Herbs that Heal.* North Adams: Storey Publishing; 2000.
- Moore M. *Medicinal Plants of the Desert and Canyon West.* Santa Fe. New Mexico: The Museum of New Mexico Press; 1989.
- Moore M. *Los Remedios: Traditional Herbal Remedies of the Southwest.* Santa Fe. New Mexico: The Museum of New Mexico Press; 1989.

- Cunningham, S. Cunningham's Encyclopedia of Magical Herbs. Woodbury: Llewellyn Publications; 2000.

- Bergner P, Becker M. *Materia Medica* Intensive Seminar. Boulder, CO: North American Institute of Medical Herbalism, Inc; 2005.
- Gladstar R. *Herbal Healing for Woman.* New York: Fireside Publishing; 1993.

Disclaimer and Reminders:

This information is presented for educational purposes only, and is in no way intended to be medical advice!

This is an introduction to a vast world of knowledge, and I encourage you to learn more, experiment, and share your findings. I hope this information inspires you to learn more and to try making tinctures at home.

Remember, we all are one, so be excellent to yourself!